List it! Activity book for dementia patients is an anti memory loss activity book for the elderly and is developed specifically for those suffering from Dementia and Alzheimers, or other elderly citizens who may be showing signs of memory loss. Unlike other elderly activity books, these pages are tailored for those at all stages of dementia. With no complex activities, and the use of simple memory recall activities that encourage the appropriate mental patterns required for memory stability. Each page is timed and counted, which allows carers to clearly see process from the start of the book to the end of the book. Although pages are not ranked in order of complexity, the repetition of pages throughout the book will allow clear patterns of improvement to be observed by family, friends and carers.

The dementia activity book was developed from insights given by neurologists, psychologists, caregivers and dementia and alzheimers patients, to only contain what is proven to work.

It is recommended that a schedule is developed with these activities, to provide further structure to the task. This may be one page a day, one each morning and night, or a number each day for consecutive days.

Name an **Animal** Beginning with the letter ...

A		**N**	
B		**O**	
C		**P**	
D		**Q**	
E		**R**	
F		**S**	
G		**T**	
H		**U**	
I		**V**	
J		**W**	
K		**X**	
L		**Y**	
M		**Z**	

Total / 26

Time

Name a **Country** Beginning with the letter ...

A		N	
B		O	
C		P	
D		Q	
E		R	
F		S	
G		T	
H		U	
I		V	
J		W	
K		X	
L		Y	
M		Z	

Total / 26

Time

Name a **Boys Name** Beginning with the letter ...

A		N	
B		O	
C		P	
D		Q	
E		R	
F		S	
G		T	
H		U	
I		V	
J		W	
K		X	
L		Y	
M		Z	

Total / 26		Time

Name a **Girls Name** Beginning with the letter ...

A		N	
B		O	
C		P	
D		Q	
E		R	
F		S	
G		T	
H		U	
I		V	
J		W	
K		X	
L		Y	
M		Z	

Total / 26

Time

Name a **Fruit** Beginning with the letter ...

A		N	
B		O	
C		P	
D		Q	
E		R	
F		S	
G		T	
H		U	
I		V	
J		W	
K		X	
L		Y	
M		Z	

Total / 26

Time

Name a **Vegetable** Beginning with the letter ...

A		N	
B		O	
C		P	
D		Q	
E		R	
F		S	
G		T	
H		U	
I		V	
J		W	
K		X	
L		Y	
M		Z	

Total / 26	Time

Name a **Food** Beginning with the letter ...

A		N	
B		O	
C		P	
D		Q	
E		R	
F		S	
G		T	
H		U	
I		V	
J		W	
K		X	
L		Y	
M		Z	

Total / 26

Time

Name a **Movie** Beginning with the letter ...

A		N	
B		O	
C		P	
D		Q	
E		R	
F		S	
G		T	
H		U	
I		V	
J		W	
K		X	
L		Y	
M		Z	

Total / 26

Time

Name a **Song** Beginning with the letter ...

A		N	
B		O	
C		P	
D		Q	
E		R	
F		S	
G		T	
H		U	
I		V	
J		W	
K		X	
L		Y	
M		Z	

Total / 26

Time

Name a **Music Artist** Beginning with the letter ...

A		N	
B		O	
C		P	
D		Q	
E		R	
F		S	
G		T	
H		U	
I		V	
J		W	
K		X	
L		Y	
M		Z	

Total / 26

Time

Name an **Actor** Beginning with the letter ...

A		**N**	
B		**O**	
C		**P**	
D		**Q**	
E		**R**	
F		**S**	
G		**T**	
H		**U**	
I		**V**	
J		**W**	
K		**X**	
L		**Y**	
M		**Z**	

Total / 26

Time

Name an **Actress** Beginning with the letter ...

A		N	
B		O	
C		P	
D		Q	
E		R	
F		S	
G		T	
H		U	
I		V	
J		W	
K		X	
L		Y	
M		Z	

Total / 26

Time

Name an **Restaurant or Food outlet** Beginning with the letter ...

A		N	
B		O	
C		P	
D		Q	
E		R	
F		S	
G		T	
H		U	
I		V	
J		W	
K		X	
L		Y	
M		Z	

Total / 26

Time

Name a **Shop** Beginning with the letter ...

A		N	
B		O	
C		P	
D		Q	
E		R	
F		S	
G		T	
H		U	
I		V	
J		W	
K		X	
L		Y	
M		Z	

Total / 26

Time

Name a **Clothing Brand** Beginning with the letter ...

A		**N**	
B		**O**	
C		**P**	
D		**Q**	
E		**R**	
F		**S**	
G		**T**	
H		**U**	
I		**V**	
J		**W**	
K		**X**	
L		**Y**	
M		**Z**	

Total / 26

Time

Name a **Sport** Beginning with the letter ...

A		N	
B		O	
C		P	
D		Q	
E		R	
F		S	
G		T	
H		U	
I		V	
J		W	
K		X	
L		Y	
M		Z	

Total / 26

Time

Name a **Hobby** Beginning with the letter ...

A		**N**	
B		**O**	
C		**P**	
D		**Q**	
E		**R**	
F		**S**	
G		**T**	
H		**U**	
I		**V**	
J		**W**	
K		**X**	
L		**Y**	
M		**Z**	

Total / 26

Time

Name a **Bird** Beginning with the letter ...

A		N	
B		O	
C		P	
D		Q	
E		R	
F		S	
G		T	
H		U	
I		V	
J		W	
K		X	
L		Y	
M		Z	

Total / 26

Time

Name a **Professional Sportsman** Beginning with the letter ...

A		**N**	
B		**O**	
C		**P**	
D		**Q**	
E		**R**	
F		**S**	
G		**T**	
H		**U**	
I		**V**	
J		**W**	
K		**X**	
L		**Y**	
M		**Z**	

Total / 26

Time

Name a **Career** Beginning with the letter ...

A		N	
B		O	
C		P	
D		Q	
E		R	
F		S	
G		T	
H		U	
I		V	
J		W	
K		X	
L		Y	
M		Z	

Total / 26

Time

Name a **Household Item** Beginning with the letter ...

A		N	
B		O	
C		P	
D		Q	
E		R	
F		S	
G		T	
H		U	
I		V	
J		W	
K		X	
L		Y	
M		Z	

Total / 26

Time

Name an **Electrical Appliance** Beginning with the letter ...

A		N	
B		O	
C		P	
D		Q	
E		R	
F		S	
G		T	
H		U	
I		V	
J		W	
K		X	
L		Y	
M		Z	

Total / 26

Time

Name a **Kitchen Item** Beginning with the letter ...

A		N	
B		O	
C		P	
D		Q	
E		R	
F		S	
G		T	
H		U	
I		V	
J		W	
K		X	
L		Y	
M		Z	

Total / 26

Time

Name a **State or City** Beginning with the letter ...

A		N	
B		O	
C		P	
D		Q	
E		R	
F		S	
G		T	
H		U	
I		V	
J		W	
K		X	
L		Y	
M		Z	

Total / 26

Time

Name a **Word** Beginning with the letter ...

A		N	
B		O	
C		P	
D		Q	
E		R	
F		S	
G		T	
H		U	
I		V	
J		W	
K		X	
L		Y	
M		Z	

Total / 26

Time

Name a **Website** Beginning with the letter ...

A		N	
B		O	
C		P	
D		Q	
E		R	
F		S	
G		T	
H		U	
I		V	
J		W	
K		X	
L		Y	
M		Z	

Total / 26

Time

Name a **Drink** Beginning with the letter ...

A		**N**	
B		**O**	
C		**P**	
D		**Q**	
E		**R**	
F		**S**	
G		**T**	
H		**U**	
I		**V**	
J		**W**	
K		**X**	
L		**Y**	
M		**Z**	

Total / 26

Time

Name a **Party Theme** Beginning with the letter ...

A		N	
B		O	
C		P	
D		Q	
E		R	
F		S	
G		T	
H		U	
I		V	
J		W	
K		X	
L		Y	
M		Z	

Total / 26

Time

Name a **TV Character** Beginning with the letter ...

A		N	
B		O	
C		P	
D		Q	
E		R	
F		S	
G		T	
H		U	
I		V	
J		W	
K		X	
L		Y	
M		Z	

Total / 26

Time

Name a **Disney Character** Beginning with the letter ...

A		N	
B		O	
C		P	
D		Q	
E		R	
F		S	
G		T	
H		U	
I		V	
J		W	
K		X	
L		Y	
M		Z	

Total / 26

Time

Name a **Dessert** Beginning with the letter ...

A		**N**	
B		**O**	
C		**P**	
D		**Q**	
E		**R**	
F		**S**	
G		**T**	
H		**U**	
I		**V**	
J		**W**	
K		**X**	
L		**Y**	
M		**Z**	

Total / 26

Time

Name a **Dog Breed** Beginning with the letter ...

A		N	
B		O	
C		P	
D		Q	
E		R	
F		S	
G		T	
H		U	
I		V	
J		W	
K		X	
L		Y	
M		Z	

Total / 26

Time

Name a **Street** Beginning with the letter ...

A		**N**	
B		**O**	
C		**P**	
D		**Q**	
E		**R**	
F		**S**	
G		**T**	
H		**U**	
I		**V**	
J		**W**	
K		**X**	
L		**Y**	
M		**Z**	

Total / 26

Time

Name a **Dinosaur** Beginning with the letter ...

A		**N**	
B		**O**	
C		**P**	
D		**Q**	
E		**R**	
F		**S**	
G		**T**	
H		**U**	
I		**V**	
J		**W**	
K		**X**	
L		**Y**	
M		**Z**	

Total / 26

Time

Name an **Exercise** Beginning with the letter ...

A		**N**	
B		**O**	
C		**P**	
D		**Q**	
E		**R**	
F		**S**	
G		**T**	
H		**U**	
I		**V**	
J		**W**	
K		**X**	
L		**Y**	
M		**Z**	

Total / 26	Time

Name a **Song or Movie Genre** Beginning with the letter ...

A		N	
B		O	
C		P	
D		Q	
E		R	
F		S	
G		T	
H		U	
I		V	
J		W	
K		X	
L		Y	
M		Z	

Total / 26

Time

Name a **Last Name** Beginning with the letter ...

A		N	
B		O	
C		P	
D		Q	
E		R	
F		S	
G		T	
H		U	
I		V	
J		W	
K		X	
L		Y	
M		Z	

Total / 26	Time

Name an **Award** Beginning with the letter ...

A		**N**	
B		**O**	
C		**P**	
D		**Q**	
E		**R**	
F		**S**	
G		**T**	
H		**U**	
I		**V**	
J		**W**	
K		**X**	
L		**Y**	
M		**Z**	

Total / 26	Time

Name an **Olympic Sport** Beginning with the letter ...

A		N	
B		O	
C		P	
D		Q	
E		R	
F		S	
G		T	
H		U	
I		V	
J		W	
K		X	
L		Y	
M		Z	

Total / 26

Time

Name an **Body Part** Beginning with the letter ...

A		**N**	
B		**O**	
C		**P**	
D		**Q**	
E		**R**	
F		**S**	
G		**T**	
H		**U**	
I		**V**	
J		**W**	
K		**X**	
L		**Y**	
M		**Z**	

Total / 26

Time

Name a **Reptile** Beginning with the letter ...

A		N	
B		O	
C		P	
D		Q	
E		R	
F		S	
G		T	
H		U	
I		V	
J		W	
K		X	
L		Y	
M		Z	

Total / 26

Time

Name a **Band** Beginning with the letter ...

A		N	
B		O	
C		P	
D		Q	
E		R	
F		S	
G		T	
H		U	
I		V	
J		W	
K		X	
L		Y	
M		Z	

Total / 26

Time

Name a **Skill** Beginning with the letter ...

A		N	
B		O	
C		P	
D		Q	
E		R	
F		S	
G		T	
H		U	
I		V	
J		W	
K		X	
L		Y	
M		Z	

Total / 26	Time

Name a **Tool** Beginning with the letter ...

A		N	
B		O	
C		P	
D		Q	
E		R	
F		S	
G		T	
H		U	
I		V	
J		W	
K		X	
L		Y	
M		Z	

Total / 26	Time

Name a **Car or vehicle** Beginning with the letter ...

A		N	
B		O	
C		P	
D		Q	
E		R	
F		S	
G		T	
H		U	
I		V	
J		W	
K		X	
L		Y	
M		Z	

Total / 26

Time

Name an **object or thing in space** Beginning with the letter ...

A		N	
B		O	
C		P	
D		Q	
E		R	
F		S	
G		T	
H		U	
I		V	
J		W	
K		X	
L		Y	
M		Z	

Total / 26

Time

Name a **biome** Beginning with the letter ...

A		N	
B		O	
C		P	
D		Q	
E		R	
F		S	
G		T	
H		U	
I		V	
J		W	
K		X	
L		Y	
M		Z	

Total / 26	Time

Name a **Zoo animal** Beginning with the letter ...

A		N	
B		O	
C		P	
D		Q	
E		R	
F		S	
G		T	
H		U	
I		V	
J		W	
K		X	
L		Y	
M		Z	

Total / 26

Time

Name an **object or thing in the ocean** Beginning with the letter ...

A		N	
B		O	
C		P	
D		Q	
E		R	
F		S	
G		T	
H		U	
I		V	
J		W	
K		X	
L		Y	
M		Z	

Total / 26

Time

Name an **room** Beginning with the letter ...

A		**N**	
B		**O**	
C		**P**	
D		**Q**	
E		**R**	
F		**S**	
G		**T**	
H		**U**	
I		**V**	
J		**W**	
K		**X**	
L		**Y**	
M		**Z**	

Total / 26

Time

www.ingramcontent.com/pod-product-compliance
Lightning Source LLC
Chambersburg PA
CBHW052041280526
45791CB00010B/3038

* 9 7 8 1 0 7 0 5 7 5 9 9 5 *